All You Need To Know About Managing Asthma

The Best Ever Natural Treatments to Help You Get Your Life Back!

All You Need To Know About Managing Asthma

Healthy Body Books

http://www.healthybodybooks.com

ISBN-13:
978-1499708806

ISBN-10:
1499708807

This document is geared towards providing exact and
reliable information in regards to the topic and issue
covered. The publication is sold with the idea that the
publisher is not required to render accounting, officially
permitted, or otherwise, qualified services. If advice is

necessary, legal or professional, a practiced individual in the profession should be ordered.

The author of this book does not dispense medical advice or prescribe the use of any technique as a form of treatment for physical, emotional, or medical problems without the advice of a physician, either directly or indirectly. The intent of the author is only to offer information of a general nature to help you in your quest for emotional, spiritual and physical well-being. In the event you use any of the information in this book for yourself, which is your constitutional right, the author and the publisher assume no responsibility for your actions. Under no circumstances will any legal responsibility or blame be held against the publisher for any reparation, damages, or monetary loss due to the information herein, either directly or indirectly.

The information herein is offered for informational purposes solely, and is universal as so. The presentation of the information is without contract or any type of guarantee assurance.

The trademarks that are used are without any consent, and the publication of the trademark is without permission or backing by the trademark owner. All trademarks and brands within this book are for clarifying purposes only and are the owned by the owners themselves, not affiliated with this document.

Table of Contents

Introduction

Are you worried you'll never be free from Asthma?

Are you sick of Asthma ruling your life?

Do you look at other people and wonder how they get through the day and why breathing seems so easy?

Is your Asthma affecting your physical health, and exercising?

Do you wish you knew how to manage your Asthma?

In this book you will discover the most up-to-date information on beating Asthma for life including:

-What is Asthma?

-Conventional Treatments

-25 Natural Treatments to Combat Asthma

-Benefits of Natural Treatments

And much more!

I want to thank you and congratulate you for buying this book, "All You Need to Know About Managing Asthma; The Best Ever Natural Treatments to Help You Get Your Life Back!"

Taking the first step is sometimes half of the battle!

I would also like to introduce myself; my name is Simone, the creator of the Healthy Body Books. My deep-seated passion for health has driven me to create these books. Something inside of me has always called out, encouraging me to write books that health-minded individuals would want to read. Health has always been a priority in my life, even when a recent change in my routine made it much more difficult to find myself.

In spite of not feeling my best (or even much like myself), I found ways to continue achieving my goals. After searching long and hard, I found that natural therapies, diets and self-help were enough to help me get things back under control. I found out that these natural remedies were doing so much for me – and I never looked back.

If you are trying to find another way to stay healthy, the Healthy Body Books are for you. If you are anything like me, you might need to find an alternative method to reach your peak. Written by experts in terms that anybody can read, these books are designed to help you identify which aspects of your life just do not seem to be working for you. You should not let anything stop you from being the person you want to be – or from living the life you want to live. This book will help you along you journey.

Good luck!

Keep up to Date with New Releases

Thank you again for buying this Book All You Need to Know About Managing Asthma; The Best Ever Natural Treatments to Help You Get Your Life Back!

I'd like to offer you the chance to stay up-to date on new books with free access to my newsletter!

You will be getting up to date information on health, fitness and diet, and also get access to getting other Healthy Body Books for free. By joining my newsletter you will be taking a big step forward in being your Healthiest Body yet!

Just visit http://www.healthybodybooks.com and get free instant access to the Healthy Body Books newsletter today!

Chapter 1 – Asthma | What Is Asthma

Asthma attacks can be really frightening and life threatening. Asthma is a common health condition among both children and adults, and is often regarded as a mysterious illness and quite frustrating to treat. The causes of asthma are often *unknown* but most of the time is attributed to hereditary factors, allergies, and sometimes to adrenal disorders too. Some herbal remedies and other natural treatments for asthma may help prevent it or alleviate its symptoms in addition to the medical treatments prescribed by your doctor.

What Is Asthma?

Asthma is generally described as the intermittent constriction of the lungs' bronchial tubes, a chronic lung and respiratory tract condition that can produce severe respiratory symptoms. Asthma is now being considered as an "inflammatory disorder" as it is typically inflammation that causes the constriction of the bronchial airways. If an asthma attack is severe enough, it can possibly kill the individual due to asphyxiation or suffocation due to lack of oxygen from the constricted airways.

Asthma Attacks

During an asthma attack, the person's lung airways become inflamed and the bronchial wall muscles tighten, after which, the attack starts to produce extra mucus thus further narrowing the air passages to the lungs. This constriction or narrowing of the bronchial

8

tubes then causes restricted airflow, shortness of breath, wheezing, and starvation of air.

Often first appearing in childhood, Asthma attacks can appear and disappear throughout a person's life without any warning. But though an ongoing condition, it is a manageable illness that can disappear in time with the proper care and treatment. Asthma can cause various symptoms such as wheezing and coughing, and may produce from mild to moderate to severe difficulties in breathing.

Symptoms of Asthma

Asthma may cause varying symptoms among different individuals but typically, the condition is marked by wheezing symptoms (especially when exhaling), coughing, choking, difficulty in breathing or breathlessness, and at times heart palpitations and accompanying panic attacks.

Causes of Asthma

Each person has different triggers that could bring about his or her asthma attack. The immediate cause of asthmatic attacks is the tightening of the muscular walls of the lung's airways due to sudden inflammation. The size of the bronchial tubes (airways) then narrows causing difficulties in breathing. Nerves control the bronchial muscles, but what specifically triggers the nerves to cause inflammation and to constrict the airways is strangely unclear.

Generally, the main triggers for asthma may include allergic reactions, fatigue, or emotional stress factors. Other common cases are induced by exercise or respiratory infections. At certain times, Asthma can occur *without* any obvious causes or triggers. Some of the most common factors that trigger Asthma are smoke, dust, molds, pollen, pet dander, food allergies, food dyes, chemical toxins, and stress.

Asthma Statistics

Asthma affects most people of all genders and ages. More than 22 million Americans today suffer from Asthma and this is in the USA alone (statistics according to the Center of Disease Control.) Among the millions of asthma sufferers, nearly 6 million are *children* (info from the National Lung and Blood Institute.) In fact according to the American Academy of Family Physicians, in the last forty years, childhood asthma has become more prevalent among children, yet according to Mayo Clinic, asthma among children can be controlled but not absolutely cured.

Fortunately throughout the world, there are already scores of conventional treatments and natural/herbal remedies to help treat or prevent Asthma. Several medical and natural cures may now be able to help minimize the symptoms of asthma in both children and adults.

Chapter 2 – Conventional Treatments for Asthma

The treatment for asthma primarily has 2 aspects: control of acute attacks and long-term management or prevention. Oftentimes the best choices for acute asthma attacks are conventional treatments, which can immediately provide relief especially during possible life-and-death situations.

For asthma attacks that are triggered by allergies, one of the best and safest treatments to use is inhaled Cromolyn Sodium. Other drugs of similar class can be inhaled too to relieve the asthma attacks. Newer drugs such as Leukotriene inhibitors are useful and effective, too, for some patients and are less toxic.

As much as possible, refrain from using asthma *inhalers that contain steroids*. Bronchodilating medications may sometimes be used *but* these are stimulants that can increase a person's sympathetic tone and trigger anxiety. At the same time, inhalation of a bronchodilator always requires Steroid inhalers immediately right after each use. Note that although effective, if the steroids in these inhalers are not absorbed into the system, they can be *unsafe* to one's health especially with long-term use.

Theophylline, a derived drug from tea, may also have a long history of use in treating asthma, however nowadays it may no longer be as safe as doctors had once thought of it. Specifically, Theophylline can cause extreme changes in a one's personality hence possibly endangering his or her mental health.

In choosing conventional methods in treating asthmatic attacks, remember that different drugs or inhalers for asthma vary greatly in efficiency and absorbability. As of this moment, the best products to use are Pulmocort (budesonide) and Flovent (fluticasone), which are both safer compared to their older varieties.

Disadvantages of Using Conventional Medications for Asthma Attacks

These medicated inhalers for asthma may work, but for long-term control and management, these conventional methods are more problematic for the 'drug dependent' asthmatic patient. These inhalers are often *addictive* as they likely cause the bronchial tubes to become constricted again when one dose of the inhaler starts to wear off. (Drugs that are sprayed into the nose for relieving nasal congestion also have the same addictive pattern.)

There are also the Allopathic drugs that are *suppressive* in nature. These treatments tend to perpetuate the condition of asthma and may reduce the chances that the asthma will naturally disappear on its own.

Oral steroids (such as Prednisone, the commonest kind) as well are highly dangerous for asthmatics. Aside from that they are also addictive, and the level of *toxicity* from their long-term use is devastating. Try to completely avoid ever going on oral steroids for treating asthma. But if you do have to take them for emergencies, get off it as soon as possible. A general rule of thumb is the less chemical medication you can take for asthma, the better.

People with chronic asthma conditions who are now aware of these side effects from conventional medications can search for *more natural* alternatives for treating asthma.

It's not that conventional asthma medications are complicated to take (since inhaling vapor or powder is obviously trickier than just swallowing a pill), and it's also neither that most of these medications are completely dangerous (or likely to cause inconvenient side effects) especially when weighed against their benefits. It is just more on the fact that we *don't have to* incorporate medications that have chemicals into our bodies when there are obviously other *more natural* alternatives.

Chapter 3 - Natural Alternatives for Treating Asthma

Natural remedies for treating asthma have already been used for so many years to help control acute asthma and alleviate its symptoms. Natural treatments for asthma attacks help reduce the intensity of the attacks as well as manage the frequency of chronic periodic asthma. (It even also helps other people with general trouble breathing.) The advantages of using natural herbal remedies for treating asthma and other lung disorders have long been repeatedly shown throughout centuries worldwide. Most probably the only possible way to effectively control asthma is through natural/herbal treatments.

What Do "Natural", "Home Remedy", and "Alternative" Methods Mean?

Ideally, "natural methods" for treating asthma means using herbs or ingredients that can normally be found in our environment (or our bodies). This means they are NOT man-made or artificial. In contrast, (most typical) conventional medicines are *chemically* prepared and manufactured by pharmaceutical companies. Sad to say, these days even so-called "natural" herbs and supplements are in fact just artificial preparations as well made by underground unregulated profit-seeking companies.

Natural methods of treatment using more or less "raw" natural ingredients can be done at home and these are called "home remedies". While most of the time these are safe, the only problem comes when they are *misused* (i.e. use of the wrong dosage, unhygienic preparations, etc.) hence, producing dangerous health effects.

As with most "alternative medicine", these are mostly natural as well and are often used as an "alternative" to traditional or conventional Western medicine. Most conventional doctors would not usually advise this approach, although in some parts of the globe, alternative methods are considered quite traditional. Many Chinese or Eastern approaches to treatment such as Acupuncture and Qi Gong are characteristically referred to as alternative medicine.

A much newer and more accurate term exists today and it's called *"integrative medicine"*. Integrative medicine acknowledges the use of natural/alternative approaches along with traditional or conventional medicine. Both can be used together – or in other words "integrated" for optimum results.

Natural methods, alternative approaches, or home remedies are just a few simple ways to treat or manage asthma better. They are best used with traditional/ conventional medicine under the supervision of a certified medical practitioner for maximum effects.

Chapter 4 – The Benefits of Using Natural Treatments for Asthma

The popularity of using natural and/or alternative remedies to help treat asthma has some good bases to it. *On their own* though, these treatments – that are often especially "advertised" for treating asthma – such as acupuncture, yoga, special breathing techniques, etc. are NOT expected to cure or control asthma especially if used *without* any physician's consent. Still, some of these methods may have some real value to them if used via *integrative approach*, or when used in combination with conventional asthma medicines.

As with all other illnesses, getting the right treatment is essential to continue living a quality life despite having pervasive asthma. It's a fact that if asthma attacks are not treated with care, there can be serious complications ahead. Unfortunately many asthma patients really don't like being restrained to daily or twice daily inhaler treatments, and not to mention being required to use supplementary rescue inhalers during emergency attacks whenever there are sudden triggers.

Naturally, nobody wants to be tied to once or twice a day maintenance treatments when all of us live such busy lives, and most asthma treatments are very expensive. This is especially true for people who don't have prescription coverage from health insurance; the treatment costs for asthma can be a real burden. Even so, the costs of NOT being able treat asthma are also even higher.

That is the main problem with expensive conventional treatments – the cost. Additionally we *never* want to *have to* routinely intake these conventional drugs, and risk becoming dependent to the chemical substances in them. This is the main reason why many people these days now seek out *more natural* alternative approaches.

Natural remedies can help reduce the severity of asthma attacks and the frequency of them recurring. They provide *no risks* to steroid exposure and dependency or addiction to the drugs.

Still, although natural remedies are relatively low risk, they are *not* recommended to *completely* subxstitute for your typical conventional treatments. Rather, it's much better if they are used as supplemental or complementary (in addition) to your usual asthma inhalers or medicines.

Conventional treatments for asthma often potentially produce unpleasant side effects and lead to drug dependency while natural/alternative treatments with herbs and other nature-based remedies can provide relief only so far as you consult your health practitioner first before using them. *Never* discontinue your use of your conventional treatments without seeking advice from your health care provider.

Chapter 5 – 25 (+) Natural Ways to Treat Asthma

If used properly natural remedies may help you manage asthma, especially if used with your conventional treatments. Below are some of the most effective natural/alternative treatments that can help ease your asthma attacks and their recurring symptoms:

Omega-3 fatty acids diet – a diet naturally rich in fatty fish such as salmon, mackerel, or codfish. These may help decrease inflammation that leads to asthma.

Apple cider Vinegar and Honey – both are highly packed with nutrients. Honey is antiviral and antibacterial which helps prevent possible triggers. Apple cider vinegar is a great detoxifier and helps strengthen the lungs, digestive system, and immune system. It helps alleviate allergies and sinus problems as well as chronic fatigue. Add 1-2 tablespoon of ACD plus 1 teaspoon Honey to one glass of water. Drink before meals, 3 times a day. During asthma attacks, place a jar of honey under your nose to help you breathe easier.

Garlic Cloves and Ginger tea – for preventing inflammation and opening the lung's airways. Boil some distilled water with Garlic cloves and Ginger. Drink 2x daily, after waking up and going to bed.

Ginger powder, Turmeric, and Black Pepper Herbal tea – Mix 1/4 teaspoon Ginger and Turmeric powder and 1/4 ground Black pepper to 1 teaspoon Molasses or Honey. Add hot water and let infuse for a few minutes and drink. Use this treatment once per day to help prevent recurring asthma.

Indian Tobacco a.k.a Lobelia – Lobelia tincture has been used throughout history by Native American Indians as an herbal remedy for respiratory conditions such as bronchitis, asthma, and pneumonia (info from the UMMC.) It is used to help clear mucus from the lungs, throat, and bronchial airways. Mix three parts Lobelia powder with one part red chili or cayenne powder. Mix with water to form a thin syrup. During acute attacks, take 20 drops by mouth and repeat every 30 minutes. Repeat 3 to 4 times. You may also take 500 to 1,000 milligram capsules or tablets of Lobelia 3 times a day to reduce inflammation caused by air pollution. Use this for NO LONGER than 2 weeks. Warning: DO NOT give Lobelia to children under 12 years old.

Eucalyptus Oil – has an anti-inflammatory property that may help ease asthma. A German study that involved 32 patients found that their use of Eucalyptus oil may have helped cause the anti-inflammatory effects among the patients. The study's findings were published in "Respiratory Medicine" dated March, 2003.

Ephedra – a perennial evergreen plant that has been used in traditional Chinese medicine for thousands of years to help treat asthma or bronchitis (info from the University of Maryland Medical Center or UMMC). Use its dried stems and leaves to make teas or extracts. They are also available in natural tablets or capsules. *Warning: Potentially lethal. DO NOT OVERDOSE with Ephedra. DO NOT use for children.*

Spiegel seeds – Mix 1 teaspoon of Spiegel seeds into a cup of hot water and drink twice a day. Over time, this treatment has been found to help improve asthma and ease its symptoms. It's highly recommended to swallow the Spiegel seeds, but you can also steep the seeds in boiling water for a few minutes then strain them out.

Caraway seeds steam inhalation therapy – to add relief during asthma attacks, boil hot water, add caraway seeds, and breathe in the steam. You may also take a quick hot shower along with this treatment to help relieve congestion. Make sure the shower is hot enough that it stimulates your skin to perspire and open your lung airways.

Butterbur herb – it has also been shown to decrease both the severity of asthma attacks as well as its frequency. Butterbur is anti-inflammatory as well as antispasmodic (muscle spasm suppressant.) Create a tea infusion with Butterbur herbs or take it as a natural supplement capsule. *Warning: Butterbur is related to ragweed, a very potent allergen. Thus if you're allergic to ragweed, you might also want to avoid Butterbur herb.*

Boswellia – a herb that is believed to help interfere with leukotrienes or the substances that help cause inflammation leading to asthma.

German chamomile tea (Matricaria recutita) – a natural antihistamine that helps prevent allergies that trigger asthma attacks. It's very gentle, yet effective. Drink 2-3 times a day.

Elderberry, in thick syrup or Sambucol lozenges – a decongestant that can relieve nasal congestion as it opens the lung's air passages typically blocked during asthma attacks.

Ipecacuanha tincture – for controlling phlegm. Use it as directed on the label. It will help reduce the overproduction of phlegm that blocks the airways during asthma attacks.

Scutellaria herb capsules – for preventing allergies causing asthma. Take 1,000 to 2,000 milligrams 3 times a day to prevent allergic reactions. *Warning: DO NOT take Scutellaria if you have diarrhea.*

Asmatica capsules (Tylophora indica) – antispasmodic, suppresses muscle spasms that constrict the lung's airways during asthma attacks. Take 400 milligrams twice a day for 2 weeks. Repeat treatment as long as symptoms persist. It can help prevent acute attacks for up to 2 weeks after treatment.

Saiboku-to tonic – a Japanese traditional herbal mixture used for treating asthma, at least, according to University of Maryland Medical Center. A study shows that intake of Saiboku-to has allowed asthma patients to take smaller doses of corticosteroids to help manage asthma. The tonic is composed of a mixture of herbs such as licorice, ginger, skullcap, and ginseng. This tonic is available at health food stores. *Warning: Some of the herbs contained in Saiboku-to cause side effects; the substances may interfere with other herbs and medicines. Consult a reliable health practitioner first before taking this tonic.*

Essential oils – the following can be used to create aromatherapy or tea infusions: Eucalyptus oil, Peppermint oil, Laurel leaf, Clary sage, Lemon extract, and Tea tree oil. Remember to use only therapeutic grade essential oils, which are safe to use for inside or outside the body. These ingredients may be used individually or as some sort of blend. *Note: There are actually essential oil suppliers that make proprietary* *blends specifically for treating asthma. Use these essential oils with caution and only as directed.*

Other methods/ alternative remedies for treating asthma:

Acupuncture – Some studies have shown that Acupuncture can significantly improve breathing and help reduce asthma attacks, ALTHOUGH studies remain uncertain.

Biofeedback or learning to control your heart rate – Biofeedback may be helpful in managing asthma but more studies are still needed to confirm its benefits.

Structured Breathing and Relaxation techniques – Often stress can trigger asthma and breathing exercises have been found to help some patients relieve their stress. Controlled breathing techniques such as the *Papworth Method* may especially help children relieve their asthma symptoms. The Papworth method consists of taking deep calm breaths from the diaphragm and through the nose. This lung muscle training also involves some *Yoga* breath control exercises (*Pranayama techniques*) for stress relief and relaxation. Another breathing method that can be used to help manage asthma is the *Buteyko Breathing Method*. It involves taking shallow breaths and letting the carbon dioxide accumulate in the airways. This is thought to help relax the muscles in the airways producing effects that are similar to bronchodilator medicines. Some studies have shown that Buteyko breathing technique may even reduce the need for asthma inhalers although there are only very few studies that help support this claim.

Eastern Disciplines such as Yoga, Qi Gong, and Tai Chi – these exercises emphasize slow, controlled breathing techniques performed with certain body movements to help relax the muscles and reduce stress. Exercising regularly using any of these methods has effects that can certainly aid people suffering from asthma most especially after taking rescue inhalers to help them calm down after having an acute attack.

Homeopathic Carbo Vegetables – also known as Carbo veg, a homeopathic remedy which may be used to as asthma treatment when the person is still conscious but feeling faint, cold and weak (according to the University of Michigan Health System). It can be used for patients with certain concomitant symptoms such as stomach upset, acid reflux, trapped gas, belching, coughing, gagging, and also vomiting. During these cases of severe asthma attacks, consult a homeopath or other homeopathy-familiar practitioner *first* before using this remedy. Homeopathic remedies are available in health food stores as well as certified online health pharmacies.

Hydrogen peroxide (H2O2) inhalation therapy – This should NOT be used without the supervision of a certified health expert. H2O2 is innately toxic.

Immunotherapy or allergy shots – a medical procedure that introduces tiny amounts or 'shots' of your allergy triggers or 'allergens' into your system. (The allergens are typically injected every week for one year or two.) The goal is to slowly build up your resistance to your allergens as they are incrementally introduced to your body. These are highly effective for eventually curing – or at least lessening – one's allergy symptoms that eventually cause asthma. Allergy shots are somewhat painful, expensive, and can take a very long time to be effective. Fortunately, *sublingual immunotherapy* or *SLIT* for short, a.k.a. 'allergy drops', have now become popular in the US. (In Europe, this immunotherapy alternative has already been used for decades.) From the word 'Sublingual', sublingual immunotherapy or allergy drops means dropping tiny amounts of your allergens 'under your tongue'. Obviously, this is a much more 'natural' and comfortable method compared to getting allergy shots or injections.

Exercise recommendations for stress or physical-strain-induced asthma:

Physical activities – Find a sport or other form of physical activity that can minimize your risks to *exercise-induced* symptoms of asthma. Tennis, baseball, softball, and golf have intermittent rest periods that can allow you to muster control of your breathing. As much as possible, avoid running outdoors during cold weather; swimming may be a much better alternative. Trivia: Some of our world's top athletes actually have exercise-induced asthma but they're still able to compete in Olympic-level sports events successfully.

Regular Exercise – Try to get used to the effects of physical activity by exercising regularly. Warm up very slowly to until you *almost* feel the "tightness" or "constriction" typically felt during asthma attacks. Then stop to stretch, or just slow down to breathe. By taking these frequent breaks during exercise, you can often stop the further development of acute asthma attacks and help you control your symptoms better. Slowly return to your normal pace of exercise after each exercise break. This frequent regular exercise may take some time and practice or getting used to but can possibly eliminate one's need for asthma inhalers or medication during asthma attacks.

The Relaxing Breath or 4-7-8 Exercise – This exercise is breath work that acts like a natural tranquilizer. But unlike tranquilizing drugs, it is subtle at first-try but gains power with succeeding repetition and practice. Use it to relieve emotional tension to prevent the onset of asthma attacks. Steps: 1) Exhale completely through your mouth (produce a 'whoosh' sound), 2) Close your mouth and inhale through your nose quietly for four seconds, 3) Next, hold your breath for seven seconds, 4) Exhale completely again through your mouth, (still with a 'whoosh' sound) for eight seconds, 5) Repeat the process by inhaling again to complete a cycle of four 4-7-8 breaths. It's normal to feel a little lightheaded at first. Do this exercise at least twice a day *only*, and *do not* do more than four cycles each time for the first month of practicing it. You can gradually extend it to eight breaths later. Remember that exhalation should take twice as long as inhalation. Once you learn to develop this technique through regular practice, it will be a very useful tool you can use to controlling your asthma better.

Other Natural relaxation techniques like guided visual imagery and progressive muscle relaxation techniques for relieving stress and reducing a person's negative response to emotional stress, which can trigger asthma.

Using any of these said methods in addition to your traditional/conventional asthma inhalers and allergy medications for asthma prevention *may* help enhance your treatment and give you greater relief and comfort. According to some stories in fact, these might even reduce your need of frequently using your rescue inhaler.

You are encouraged to explore the hundreds of other great natural remedies for asthma to see which one might work or might work *best* for you. Who knows, you might even find relief from a *strong cup of coffee*!

Chapter 6 – Safety Precautions in Treating Asthma Naturally

Just a few considerations when it comes to treating asthma naturally...

With all the newly discovered natural remedies and medicines out there today, people wonder if experts have already discovered a real natural cure for asthma. Unfortunately, Asthma still cannot be cured one hundred percent by any type of treatment. In fact experts say that asthma medicines or supplements that claim they can cure Asthma must be avoided at all cost. Be wary of those medicines that 'doctors' prescribe to permanently cure your asthma.

You may be bothered by your serious asthma attacks and be tempted to try and explore some so-called "alternative" remedies such as special diets, vitamin supplements, cytotoxicity testing and others. Though these solutions may sound very promising, the bad news is that the chances of curing your asthma are very low. Often, these are just false-claims treatments that only go for profit.

How to Evaluate the Claims of Alternative Therapies

To evaluate commercial claims of what certain natural/ herbal products can really do, look for scientific-based sources of info that will help you prove or dispute their claims.

If so, in case you have decided to try using certain natural/alternative methods or other medicines to cure your asthma, or in this sense any other illnesses, make sure that you first carefully weigh the risks and benefits you can get out of it. You must NEVER stop taking your asthma medicines in favor of any alternative treatment without consulting your doctor first.

You must also be very cautious in adding herbs and natural supplements to your treatment because some of them can interact negatively with your medicines. Consult your doctor first.

There is a website called RVita.com and you can get facts in there about the most reliable alternative treatments you can use. RVita provides a user-friendly chart on their site for each therapy that is reputed to help a person with certain conditions. The chart indicates the therapies' proven effectiveness.

Due to the non-regulation of natural/alternative asthma remedies available these days, it's very hard to know which kinds of remedies to get. As basic precaution, it is highly advisable to observe the following steps in trying out other forms of treatment:

1. Consult your doctor first before trying any remedy for asthma. Some herbs or dietary supplements may interact negatively with other drugs/medications or other natural substances.

2. If you experience side effects like vomiting, rashes, nausea, palpitation, insomnia and anxiety, stop using your herbal product right away and report the side effects to your doctor.

3. Carefully select the brands that you plan to use. Only purchase products from brands that properly list their ingredients (the herb's common and scientific names), dosage guidelines, and expiration date. The potential side effects must also be clearly indicated. Other information to look for is the name and address of their manufacturer as well as batch and lot number.

Many herbs and natural supplements are still not tested or may not have been thoroughly tested yet so you must be very careful and consult your doctor first before considering them. Some herbs may trigger an attack and may even worsen your current condition. For instance, some natural supplements come with bee pollen that may trigger your asthma if you are somewhat allergic to pollen.

Some herbs that have been discovered to treat asthma have also been found to interact adversely with other drugs. For example, ginkgo biloba, which helps to decrease the inflammation in one's lungs have been discovered to cause bleeding problems in some people taking Coumadin as their blood thinner. Another example is Licorice Root, which helps soothe the lungs of people suffering from asthma attacks. It can cause tremendous increase in blood pressure. Ephedra had once been used quite popularly as a bronchodilator but it is no longer recommended these days due to its serious side effects including possible death.

If you have any doubts about any natural supplement or alternative remedy regarding its claims or possible side effects, call your health care provider and ask for advice before   actually   taking   them.

Chapter 7 – Managing Asthma: Long-Term Control and Prevention

Even though there's no 100% proven natural cure for asthma yet, it cannot be denied that its symptoms can be controlled and prevented using the right combination of asthma medications.

To help in the proper management of asthma, your goal is to:

Get a correct and accurate asthma diagnosis from a certified physician or health care provider.

Seek advice and medication for treating coexisting conditions that can worsen you asthma symptoms, such as allergic rhinitis, GERD (acid reflux disease), and sinusitis.

Work with your physician to develop the best asthma action plan treatment for you.

Keep an asthma diary for recording all your symptoms and medication use and for tracking down every possibility that you will get an attack.

Avoid all triggers or possible causes of your asthma, including outdoor irritants such as smoke, air pollution, or smog. Also remember to always keep a clean house.

Medicate before doing any strenuous physical activities to prevent exercise-induced asthma.

Exercise daily to strengthen fitness and maintain your normal weight.

Get enough sleep or plenty of opportunities to relax and ease stress.

Eat healthy nutritious foods to maximize your immunity.

Observe a proper diet that is especially customized for asthmatics.

Call your health care provider immediately upon any sign of asthma symptoms.

Get regular check-ups for breathing tests to make certain that your asthma is well-managed as well as to know whether your medications are still working optimally.

Research traditional Chinese medicine and Ayurvedic treatments (traditional Indian healing system) and try to find out whether any of these systems may possibly offer you significant help along with your conventional meds, special diet, and herbal/natural treatments.

Reminder:

Integrative asthma treatments combining traditional/conventional medicines with natural/alternative therapies DO have a place in possibly curing and alleviating the symptoms of asthma. Although, they CANNOT totally replace you asthma medicine or inhalers; use them only in addition to your current treatments for the best results.

Always observe proper dosage and seek medical advice before trying out any new remedies. Trust your physician or certified health care provider to give you the proper guidance you would always need in managing both your acute attacks and chronic/recurring asthma.

Lastly, take responsibility for keeping your lifestyle healthy. Perform breathing exercises regularly along with your other proven healthy self-care measures for preventing or lessening the severity of your illness. You hold the key to living your life better with Asthma.

Steps to Success Action Plan

Steps to Success has been put together to give you somewhere to start on getting your Asthma under control. Asthma can control your life but by making a start and taking your life in your own hands you'll be one step closer to living in harmony in your life.

To really have success you may need to use this action plan a few times and trial a few different things to get the result you're after. Test, Measure and Monitor needs to become your motto until your Asthma is under control again.

Step 1- Accept that Asthma is affecting your life!

Step 2- Grab a notebook or start a diary to monitor your progress. This is a journey; note everything that sets of your Asthma as you may have ups and downs. By having notes to refer you find it much easier to keep track of what is working and what isn't.

Step 3 –Make a commitment to work on your Asthma. Decide which natural treatments you are going to try, and make you try each treatment a couple of times to test how well it works for you. Not every Treatment will work for everyone, making sure you find the one that works for you may be a journey, but it will be worth it!

Step 4- Monitor yourself for 3 weeks and see how you go. If the desired result has not been achieved please go back and see if there is anything else you could do, or add to your daily tasks that would improve your results.

There may be something you are doing that isn't helping, so swap it out for something else.

Conclusion

Thank you again for reading this book!

I hope this book was able to help you to fully understand Asthma, and what you can be doing to improve the quality of your life! Taking control of Asthma means having a healthy body and that is something to aim for!

The next step is to put this knowledge to good use and attempt to get the healthy body you have always dreamed off, you are off to a flying start by reading this book and taking advantage of the Action Plan included.

Finally, if you enjoyed this book, please take the time to share your thoughts and post a review on Amazon. It'd be greatly appreciated!

Thank you and good luck!

Bonus Chapter

This Bonus Chapter is from the book Are You Sick Of Your Allergies Yet? The Only Book You'll Ever Need to Eliminate Your Allergies for Life! Enjoy!

Spring Allergies

Now that you know a few methods for treating spring allergies, also known as seasonal allergic rhinitis and hay fever, there are a few more things you should understand about avoiding common causes of the problem. More than 35 million Americans experience hay fever every year, but by steering clear of the problem they might also have the opportunity to avoid sniffles and sneezes.

The biggest cause of spring allergies is pollen. Pollen is not all bad. In fact, pollen significantly helps plant fertilization. On the downside, pollen also gets into the nose of an allergic person's nose and wreaks havoc on his or her immune system.

Pollen is such a nuisance because it travels quite a bit. In fact, one piece of pollen can travel miles at a time. More pollen in the air means more unnecessary symptoms. Fortunately, there are tools available that allow you to track the amount of pollen in your area. Local weather forecasts and the website for the American Academy of Allergy, Asthma and Immunology are both incredibly helpful.

Plants to Avoid

Of course, there is no escaping some of these plants. If you can size up potential problems, you might have a better shot at eliminating seasonal allergy symptoms from your life.

Avoid trees like ash, beech, juniper, palm, willow, maple and elm. These culprits spread pollen that leads to a runny nose and constant sniffles.

Certain weeds and grasses are also frequent spreaders of pollen. These include salt grass, sweet vernal and Bermuda grass.

Avoiding these plants could be difficult for you if you live in one of the worst cities for pollen. In fact, these American locations are all over states like Tennessee, Kentucky, Louisiana, Virginia and Texas. The Midwest isn't exactly safe either – these areas are no strangers to pollen.

Though most seasonal allergies strike during the spring, it is important that you remain vigilant during other seasons as well. You should avoid doing tasks like raking leaves without proper gear. Stirring up leaves makes it quite easy for you to experience a reaction.

Understand the Weather

Coping with seasonal allergies also requires you to pay attention to the weather outside. Days with lots of wind cause more allergies, as the breeze tends to carry pollen. You will have better luck going outside on (and right after) rainy days.

Symptoms

The symptoms of spring allergies are not much unlike those for other types of allergies. You may experience a runny nose or constantly watery eyes. You may find yourself sneezing and coughing frequently. Sometimes the symptoms manifest in the form of itchy eyes that develop dark circles underneath. For some people, spring allergies are related to asthma.

Spring Allergy Diagnosis

Your doctor may suggest you speak to an allergist to complete testing for spring allergies. The most common form of diagnosis is a skin test. The doctor will inject a small amount of allergen under the skin, usually on the back. If you are allergic to the allergen the doctor has injected, a small hive will develop.

In some cases, the allergist will proceed with a radioallergosorbent test also known as an RAST. This is a blood test used to determine the levels of antibody in your system. The test may show that while you are sensitive to certain allergens, you are not necessarily going to exhibit the full range of allergic symptoms.

Upon learning that you do have spring allergies, the doctor may prescribe a medication or encourage you to look into the natural remedies mentioned in this book.

Prevent Mold

Mold is a major component of allergies. If you are trying to be allergy-free this season, take the following measures to prevent mold from growing in your home:

- Ensure that water is not getting stopped in your yard. You may require landscaping to have a slope built leading away from your house.
- Ensure that your rain gutters are taking water away from your house. A poor gutter system is responsible for plenty of moisture that might build up in your home.
- Check your basement on a regular basis for water and forms of moisture.
- Always turn on your bathroom fan when you take a shower. Mold grows when the fan is not turned on.

More Tips for Avoiding Spring Allergies

These tips will also help you avoid allergies:

- Avoid parking your car under trees and near bushes. When allergy season is in full bloom you do not want to go anywhere near these guys.
- Keep your home cool with an air conditioner in addition to a dehumidifier. This will prevent molds and pollens from interfering with your system. You should keep the air in your home dry at all costs.
- Never wear your shoes inside the house. This tracks pollen inside.
- Change your clothes as soon you come home from being outside. Better yet, take a shower after you spend any time outside.
- While many people are against using harsh chemicals like bleach, it is a highly effective means of eliminating allergen proteins from your home. Bleach breaks down these allergens, preventing symptoms altogether even when it is diluted with water. Spray the diluted solution onto furniture, carpets and counters.

Spring allergies are no walk in the park – literally. You might not be able to visit your favorite places or even walk outside any time of the year. With a few changes, you can live comfortably without the threat of spring allergies.

To check out the rest of this book "Are You Sick Of Your Allergies Yet? The Only Book You'll Ever Need to Eliminate Your Allergies for Life!" Just log on to Amazon. com

Other Books you may be interested in...

Below you'll find some of my other books currently available through Amazon. Healthy Body Books now has over 30 books in the series, so jump on line and check them out today!

Stop Snoring: Proven Techniques to Stop You Snoring Once and For All!

Exercise for Weight loss: 50 Tips to a Happier, Healthier You!

The Ultimate Guide to Being Fit for Life: Take Control of your Body and Transform your Life!

The Beginners Guide to Alternative Therapies: The Top 10 Types of Alternative Therapies Explained!

You can simply search for these amazing titles on the Amazon website.

Free Gift

Thank you again for buying this Book, All You Need to Know About Managing Asthma; The Best Ever Natural Treatments to Help You Get Your Life Back!

I'd like to reward you with this by offering you free access to my newsletter!

You will be getting up to date information on health, fitness and diet, and also get access to getting other Healthy Body Books for free. By joining my newsletter you will be taking a big step forward in being your Healthiest Body yet!

Just visit http://www.healthybodybooks.com and get free instant access to the Healthy Body Books newsletter today!

Lastly once you finish reading this book would please review this book on Amazon. With your feedback I continue to make this book better and better.

Thank you

Printed in Great Britain
by Amazon